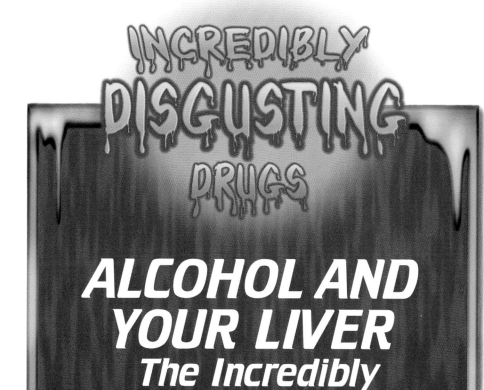

ALCOHOL AND YOUR LIVER
The Incredibly Disgusting Story

Theresa Anne Booley

the rosen publishing group's
rosen central
new york

Dedicated to
Morris and Tara Seletta,
Maia Plimpton,
and Robert Andrew Ganoush

Published in 2000 by The Rosen Publishing Group, Inc.
29 East 21st Street, New York, NY 10010

Library of Congress Cataloging-in-Publication Data

Booley, Theresa Anne.
    Alcohol and your liver : the incredibly disgusting story /
Theresa Anne Booley.
       p. cm.— (Incredibly disgusting drugs)
    Includes bibliographical references and index.
    Summary: Discusses alcohol, emphasizing its damaging physiological effects on the mind and body, most especially the liver.
    ISBN 0-8239-3254-0
    1. Alcohol abuse—Juvenile literature. [1. Alcohol abuse.] I. Title.
II. Series.

 2000
616.8—dc21

Manufactured in the United States of America

CONTENTS

Introduction: There's a First Time for Everything

When Horatio's parents went out one Friday night, some of his friends from his eighth-grade homeroom class came over. It was the same crowd he always hung out with: Tonya, the basketball player; Ezra, Horatio's best friend since fifth grade; Winston and Heath, the twins; and Lorella, who had just arrived at the school in September. Winston and Heath were video game experts. That seemed to be all they ever did and all they ever talked about. They hogged up the joysticks until Horatio and the others got bored waiting for a turn to play.

"Well, this is great," said Tonya, looking exasperated. Winston cheered as he finished the next level of the video game.

"Like, are they ever going to finish playing?" asked Lorella.

"Hey, what is this stuff in the cabinet?" called Ezra, who had wandered into the kitchen. He came back with a big bottle of rum. *"We don't have this stuff at our house."*

"Oh, that's rum," Horatio replied. *"My parents drink it sometimes."*

"Yeah, mine, too!" said Lorella. *"Tastes gross! Let's try it anyway!"*

Tonya and Ezra looked as if they wanted to try it, too. The twins were too hypnotized by the video game to hear what was going on, and everybody ignored them.

Horatio didn't know what to do; he'd never tasted alcohol himself and he had a feeling he wasn't supposed to, but it was kind of tempting! He felt a little bit scared, but his friends looked really eager to open the bottle. *"Come on, Horatio, we just want to try the stuff!"* said Tonya. *"Hey, dude, don't be a wimp,"* Ezra said.

"OK, I'll try it, too," Horatio said. Ezra opened the bottle and took a sip of the rum. He passed it around to Tonya and Lorella, who each drank a little bit from the bottle. None of them looked quite sure whether they liked the taste or not.

Horatio took the bottle from Lorella and took a big gulp. It tasted so strong! There was a burning feeling all the way to his stomach as the alcohol made its way down. It made his eyes water, and he started coughing.

Soon the four of them had passed the bottle around several times, taking little sips each time. Horatio's throat was still burning, and he felt a little woozy, as if he had just woken up after a long nap and wasn't quite sure what time it was. The level of rum in the bottle was falling, and Horatio hoped his parents wouldn't find out. Horatio started to feel light and silly, and suddenly wasn't worrying much about anything. Tonya put on some music and everybody started dancing wildly. As he leaped around the room, Horatio felt like he could hardly control his body. Somebody knocked over a vase of dried flowers that had been given to Horatio's mom a long time ago. They all ran outside and ran through the garden, making lots of noise. Then they came back inside to dance some more. It was so much fun.

Two hours later, Lorella was in the bathroom watching Horatio puke into the toilet. Horatio felt horrible. The alcohol had made him feel wonderful for a little while, but then the room had started spinning and he had begun to feel nauseous. Really nauseous. Horatio had become so sick *to his stomach that he had run to the bathroom and stood over the toilet with tons of brown puke spilling out of his mouth. He could see pieces of the macaroni and cheese he had eaten for dinner landing in the toilet. He was dizzy. His head hurt. He wanted to cry. He promised himself that he would never, ever drink alcohol again. Lorella looked pretty grossed out by the whole scene, and suddenly she was vomiting in the bathroom sink.*

There were sounds at the front door, and Horatio's parents stepped into the house. Uh-oh. "We're home!" they said.

This book is all about alcohol and its effects on your body—especially your liver and your brain. Alcohol is a drug, just like cocaine and marijuana. Because many people drink alcohol, and because alcohol is legal, it is easy to think that alcohol is less dangerous than other drugs. That's not true. As we will see, alcohol is a very dangerous substance, especially when people use it irresponsibly!

1 Alcohol: The Basics

So you think you know what alcohol is, huh? It's that stuff that gets people drunk, right?

Actually, there are hundreds of alcohols. Almost all of them are toxic (poisonous) chemicals that definitely do not make you drunk. Methanol (which is found in products like hairspray, aftershave, and nail-polish remover) can cause blindness and horrendous brain damage after a few sips. Antifreeze contains another alcohol that can quickly make people extremely ill. Paint thinner is another product that contains dangerous alcohols. These kinds of alcohols are not anything you would want to drink—they are extremely poisonous.

The kind of alcohol that people drink is called ethyl alcohol, or ethanol. It isn't as toxic as the other alcohols, but it is still a poison! Beer, wine, whiskey, rum, vodka, tequila, and gin are just a few kinds of alcoholic beverages. In this book, when we talk about alcohol, we're really talking about all of these drinks that contain ethanol.

Alcohol is made by a process known as fermentation. In fermentation, tiny microorganisms turn sugar into ethanol. The sugar comes from whatever food substance the drink is being made from. In wine, the sugar comes from grapes. In rum, the sugar comes from sugarcane. In vodka, the sugar comes from potatoes. Other alcoholic beverages might use the sugar from wheat, apricots, or plums.

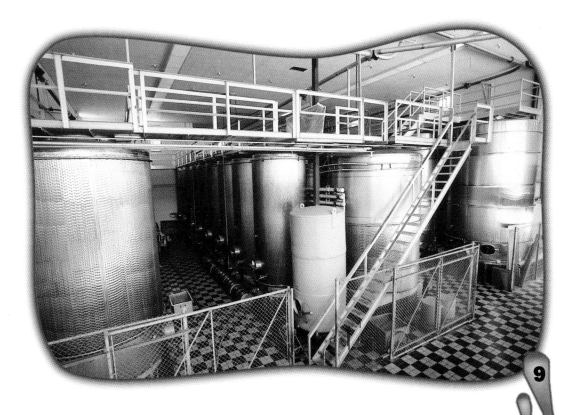

Alcoholic beverages contain different amounts of alcohol. Beer is about 6 percent alcohol. Wine has about 15 percent alcohol. Some "hard" alcoholic drinks such as vodka or rum can be more than 60 percent alcohol! The percentage of alcohol in a beverage is sometimes referred to as a drink's proof. A drink's proof is twice its alcohol content. A beverage that is 90 proof, for example, contains 45 percent alcohol.

WHO DRINKS ALCOHOL?

In the United States, nine out of ten adults drink alcohol. At some point in their life, half of all Americans will have a problem caused by alcohol. About one in every ten adults will suffer from the serious disease called alcoholism.

Alcohol is not always bad. Most people who drink alcohol are not alcoholics. Many people enjoy the taste of beer, wine, and other kinds of alcohol, although many others dislike the taste. But alcohol can be very dangerous. It can do INCREDIBLY DISGUSTING things to your body—to your liver, brain, and almost every other organ in your body—and it can make people die much too early.

So if alcohol is so dangerous, why do so many people drink? Well, besides the taste, the main thing that people like about ethanol is that it can make them drunk. Feeling drunk is not the same for everybody. Some people become happy and talkative; many others feel sad, tired, angry, or even violent. Many people drink alcohol to avoid the problems in their life, or to "loosen up" so that they feel more relaxed and happy when they party, or to feel less shy around other people. But using alcohol is not so simple because alcohol does not always make people feel good.

So what's it like being drunk?

Some people enjoy the feeling. Drunkenness can make shy people bolder, and it can help unhappy people to temporarily forget their worries. Some people say that getting drunk makes them happier or helps them have a great time. But let's look a little more closely at what it means to be drunk.

Alcohol lowers a person's inhibitions—controls over thoughts, feelings, and behavior. This is why alcohol so often makes people act in uncharacteristic ways. Drunk people are less able to control their behavior. They may be

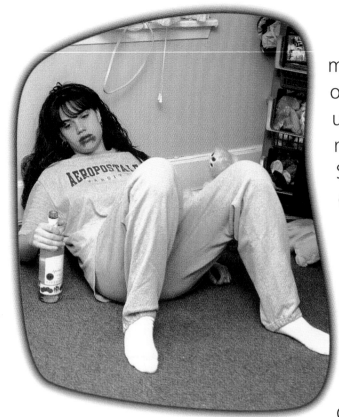

more prone to get angry or fight, or to act out sexually in ways they would not if they were sober. Shy people may find it easier to talk to other people, although alcohol makes some people morose or withdrawn in certain situations. Though this lessening of control is a reason why lots of teens like to drink, alcohol is actually a depressant, meaning that it acts to slow down, or depress, the body's systems.

Alcohol can make you feel sad or low in energy. Alcohol also slows down your thinking power and your reflexes, which is why drinking and driving is such a terrible idea. People can quickly start to lose their balance, to slur their words, and to vomit when they drink too much. Some have blackouts, which means that they lose all memory of where they were or what they did for long periods of time while drunk. People who keep on drinking beyond this point often pass out (become unconscious) or even die.

What about people who get drunk every day?

Alcoholics are people who are addicted to alcohol. Alcoholism is a chronic (long-lasting) disease with a deadly progression over many years. A person can be drunk without being an alcoholic, and an alcoholic is not always drunk. Alcoholics frequently suffer negative long-term consequences from their addiction. These can include severe mental and physical health problems, legal and financial difficulties, and troubled personal relationships. But remember that although getting drunk or misusing alcohol once or just a couple of times does not mean you are an alcoholic, there can be tremendously damaging consequences from even one such incident. It takes

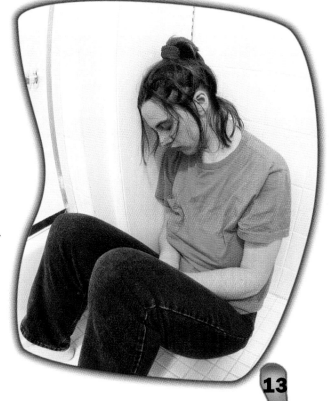

only one miscalculation behind the wheel of a car to change a lot of lives for the worse, forever. Or one night of unprotected sex while under the influence of alcohol to destroy all your hopes for the future.

Drinking responsibly?
What do you mean?

You need to be twenty-one years old to drink legally in the United States, and—although many people start drinking before that age—it's a good idea to wait until you're an adult before you decide whether or not you want to use alcohol. Drinking responsibly means drinking legally, in a safe place, without getting so drunk that you lose control. But nobody really needs to drink, although that's something Horatio has yet to learn.

2 Drunk Driving: An Incredibly Stupid Idea

Horatio was now nineteen, but he had not gotten any smarter about alcohol. That party back in eighth grade was the first time he and his buddies had ever gotten drunk, but it wasn't the last! Every weekend he would party with his buddies, and that meant plenty of beer and plenty of friends. One night around Christmas, Horatio and his girlfriend, Lorella, drove in her parents' car to a party at the Squealing Eel, the coolest club in town. When they got there, almost everyone was drunk. The party was full of energy, and there were people everywhere. After two beers and two shots of hard liquor, Horatio and Lorella were both feeling really "loose" and excited.

Lorella's beeper went off, and she went to the pay phone to make a call. When she came

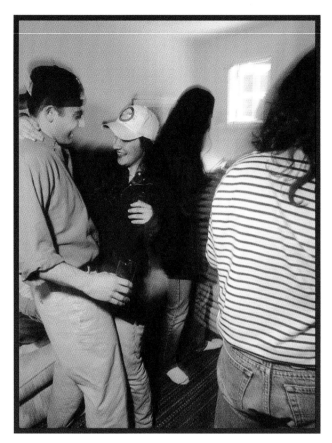

back, she said, "Hey, Horatio, Ana Maria is having a party now, too! Let's go! She's inviting us!" Ana Maria was Lorella's best friend from high school.

"OK, Lorella, let's go after we have one more drink!" said Horatio, and he went to get more beer. At the bar, their friends Mike and Eliana staggered over. They looked totally wasted. They had been playing drinking games at the bar, and each of them had drunk at least eight beers.

The kids went outside into the cold air and got into the car. Horatio did the driving. He drove out of the parking lot onto the road and sped away.

Horatio was too drunk to drive, but nobody in the car noticed. Everybody was too drunk to notice. The car wobbled from one side of the road to the other. Horatio was going 65, 75, 85 miles an hour, swerving around turns, honking his horn whenever a car passed in the other direction. Horatio was so busy laughing and talking that he barely looked at the road in front of him.

CRASH! When the car hit the big oak tree on the sidewalk, a huge noise echoed through the freezing night. Lorella and Eliana went flying through the windshield.

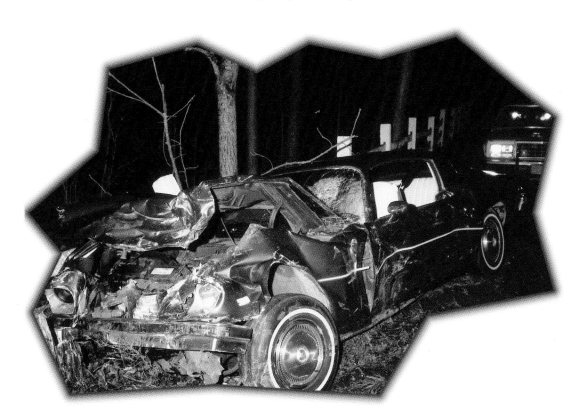

Lorella hit the trunk of the tree headfirst and died in a milli-second. Eliana tumbled down into a ditch and lay still in a pool of mud. Neither Mike nor Horatio saw any of this because they were both bleeding and had been knocked unconscious. A minute later somebody passed by and saw the wrecked car. Ambulances soon came to rescue the kids.

Mike died after a week in the intensive care unit of the hospital. Eliana survived, but with terrible brain damage. She needed to learn how to walk again.

Horatio was the luckiest. He woke up a few hours later, in the hospital, with two broken legs and a whole lot of cuts, aches, and bruises. The police were waiting to talk with him.

The moral of this story is pretty simple. Drinking alcohol makes driving an extremely dangerous game. Never, ever drive under the influence of alcohol. You should know that one of the main causes of death among teenagers is drunk-driving accidents. More teens die from auto accidents than from cancer, AIDS, or suicide. So when you get your license to drive, make sure to promise yourself that you will never drive drunk.

If you are in a situation where alcohol is being used and you have to travel in a car, make sure that there is a designated driver. Choosing someone to stay sober, and relying only on that person to do all the driving for the night, is the best way to prevent a deadly accident. Because young people often feel pressured by their friends and peers to drink, it can be hard to be a designated driver. So remember that designated drivers are there for the safety of the group and that they are avoiding alcohol so that their friends can drink responsibly. Never try to tempt a designated driver with alcohol!

3 Alcohol and Your Liver: A Bad Combination

How does alcohol work? How does it make people drunk?

Great question! Would you believe that nobody knows exactly how alcohol makes people drunk? Scientists are still trying to figure that question out. They believe that alcohol seeps into the brain and loosens up the membranes that surround your brain cells. Those membranes start acting differently, which makes the whole brain act abnormally. Gross! An abnormal brain? That does not sound good!

It sure doesn't! It sounds pretty scary. Why would I ever want to mess around with my brain? And how does it get to my brain, anyway?

When people drink, alcohol gets absorbed from their stomachs and small intestines into

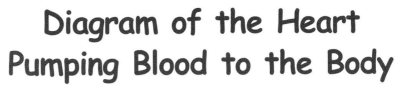

Diagram of the Heart
Pumping Blood to the Body

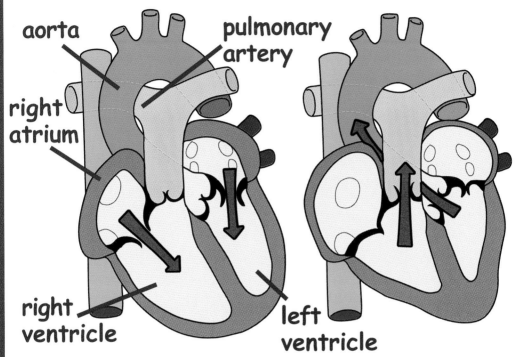

aorta

pulmonary artery

right atrium

right ventricle

left ventricle

Blood enters the ventricles, the large chambers, which close and pump blood through the pulmonary artery, which conveys venous blood to the lungs and the aorta, which separates into branch arteries that carry blood throughout the body.

their bloodstreams. Blood, pumped by the heart, flows to every part of the body—the brain, the liver, the toes, everywhere! When binge drinkers drink too much too fast, they can become unconscious or even die suddenly. Alcoholics can get horrible health problems from drinking all the time, and die slowly over years and years. Let's look at what alcohol does to your body and at some of the most disgusting diseases you can get from drinking too much alcohol.

We'll start with your liver because that's one of the most important organs that can get sick. But we won't forget to talk about the brain, the heart, and other cool places in your body that can be destroyed by alcohol.

healthy liver

The liver is the body's organ responsible for important changes in many of the substances contained in the blood.

ALCOHOL AND YOUR LIVER

What's a liver?

Have you seen liver in the supermarket or on your dinner plate? You have a nice big liver yourself, on the right side of your belly (it's a lovely reddish brown, smooth, soft, and as healthy as can be). If you relax your belly muscles, you may be able to feel the edge of your liver on the right just underneath your ribs.

What does your liver do?

The answer is pretty simple: The liver's main job is to remove poisons from the body. The liver is like a big, complicated sponge. Blood flows through tiny blood vessels in the liver, and the liver absorbs the poisons in the blood. Then it converts the poisons into safe chemicals and sends them out to your small intestine. It sends them there in the form of a liquid called bile. Bile is a completely yucky yellow liquid that gets made every day by your liver.

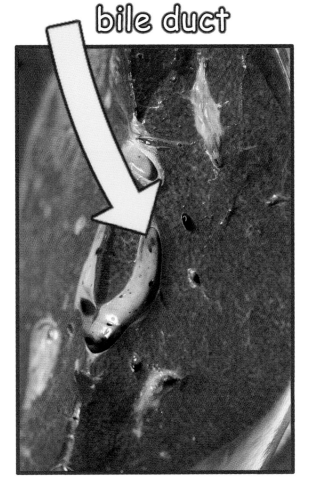

bile duct

Bile ducts transport bile, a fluid secreted by the body to aid in the absorption of fats, from the liver to the duodenum, or small intestine.

Now that you know about livers and bile, let's look at what alcohol can do to your liver. When you drink alcohol, it gets absorbed into your bloodstream and quickly reaches the liver. A little bit of alcohol is quickly sucked up into the liver and broken down into safe chemicals, and the rest goes to the brain and the rest of the body. What happens if you drink lots of alcohol? The liver can only break down a little bit of alcohol at a time, and the extra alcohol stays around in the bloodstream, which means people get more drunk and stay drunk for a longer time! Most livers can handle about one alcoholic drink every half-hour, which is why you should not drink large amounts of alcohol quickly. The cells of the liver can also become tired out, and then they start relying on less efficient ways of breaking down alcohol. That's when your liver can start to get sick.

One of the coolest things about livers is that they can regenerate, or grow back, parts of themselves that get damaged. Most of your body cannot regenerate—can you imagine somebody growing back a finger, a nose, or a brain? Because the liver has the talent to regenerate, when it gets damaged it can sometimes recover. But not always.

Tell me something else incredibly fascinating about livers!

Fatty liver is the first sign that the liver is unable to cope with the amount of alcohol it needs to break down. Fatty liver is not a permanent thing, but it's a sign that your liver cannot keep up with all of the alcohol. It happens as soon as you drink a large amount of alcohol and lasts for about a week afterward. Your liver changes from a beautiful shiny reddish brown to a dull, greasy, yellowish, gooey appearance. It can get really big and painful. Under the microscope you can see lots of fat stuck in the liver cells.

Fortunately, fatty liver goes away when people stop drinking, and it isn't really dangerous on its own. But it's a warning sign to stop drinking, and it is pretty gross-looking!

Tell me something even worse!

Alcohol hepatitis is the next bad thing to happen to your liver. Alcohol hepatitis is pretty awful, and it happens mainly to people who have been drinking heavily for a few years. Hepatitis means "swollen liver," and that is exactly what happens in this disease.

Alcohol slowly kills liver cells, and when enough liver cells die the whole liver itself gets

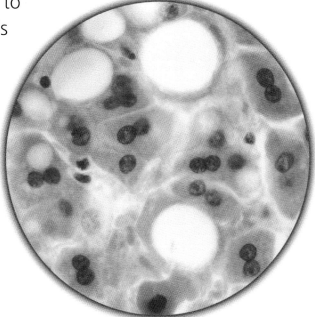

Acute alcohol hepatitis, or inflammation of the liver caused by chronic alcohol abuse, can be cured only if the sufferer stops drinking.

jaundice

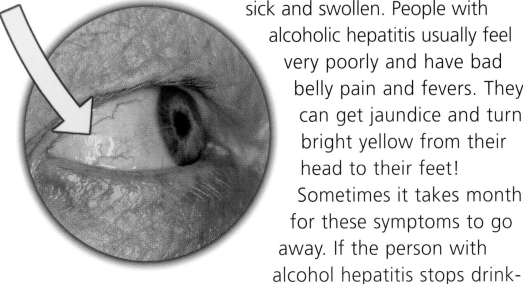

This man has jaundiced eyes, often the result of alcohol hepatitis. Jaundice is frequently caused by the obstruction, or blockage, of the body's bile ducts.

sick and swollen. People with alcoholic hepatitis usually feel very poorly and have bad belly pain and fevers. They can get jaundice and turn bright yellow from their head to their feet! Sometimes it takes months for these symptoms to go away. If the person with alcohol hepatitis stops drinking, he or she usually gets better after a while, but by definition an alcoholic finds it very difficult, if not impossible, to stop drinking.

Cirrhosis is permanent liver damage. Alcoholism can cause cirrhosis. Cirrhosis is a terrible disease because everyone needs a healthy liver.

Remember the beautiful, smooth, reddish brown liver of nondrinkers? Well, cirrhosis turns that lovely liver into the ugliest thing you've ever seen! Livers with cirrhosis are packed with tough, stringy scar tissue. A few knobby lumps of new liver desperately try to regenerate, but they are too sick to handle more alcohol. These livers are bumpy, small, and hard—and they can turn awful shades of green because of bile. A liver with cirrhosis is really not a pleasant sight.

Believe it or not, cirrhosis can be even more incredibly disgusting than that. Not only is your liver a shrunken, knobby, green lump that's sickening to look at, but it doesn't work well at all. That means that alcohol and other harmful chemicals can float around in your body without being removed by the liver. Some of these chemicals make people's brains get so sick that they don't know where they are or who their friends are.

Another problem that people with cirrhosis can have is fluid filling up their bellies. This condition is called ascites. A person can become very sick if the liver can't

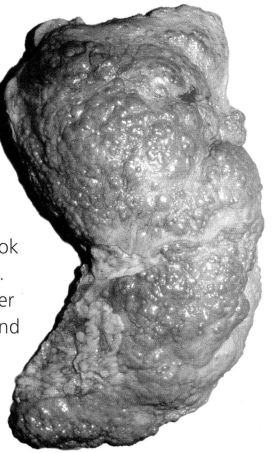

Cirrhosis is the severe disruption of normal liver function, caused by the growth of nodules—abnormal, knobby protuberances—on the liver. The cause of cirrhosis is almost always long-term alcohol abuse, hepatitis, or both.

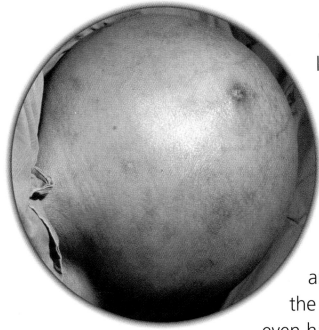

handle all of the pressure from the blood that the rest of the body sends to it. Doctors drain the fluid with a long needle. The liver can fill up with gallons of fluid.

One of the worst things that liver cirrhosis can cause is bleeding in your esophagus. Your esophagus is the tube that connects your mouth and your stomach. Because the liver is so sick, it can't even handle the blood that gets sent to it. The blood sits around in your veins, waiting to get to the liver—like a backed-up sink. Sometimes these backed-up veins are visible on the surface of the skin, looking like big blue spaghetti strands all over the belly. But watch out! One of the veins in the esophagus can weaken, swell up, and burst!

That is a real disaster: Blood starts pouring into the esophagus, and then you start to vomit bright red blood!

(Are you grossed out yet?) It is very hard to cure people with esophageal bleeding. They are already sick from all the alcohol, and they bleed very fast. Often they die quickly from the loss of blood. This is one of the most tragic ways in which alcoholics get sick and die.

Finally, there is cancer. Cancer is a disease that happens when cells in some part of your body (intestines, breast, skin, liver, or any other part) start to grow uncontrollably. It usually makes a tumor—a growing lump—and sometimes the tumor can spread all over the body. Liver cancer is one of the most deadly cancers of all. Alcoholics get liver cancer ten times more often than ordinary people! They also get a lot of cancer of the mouth, esophagus, and stomach.

Alcohol is just as harmful to other organs, too. In the next chapter we'll look at the dangerous effects of alcohol on other parts of your body.

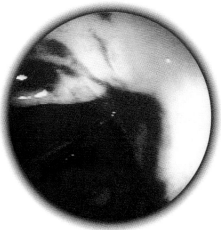

A bleeding esophagus, caused by cancer. Alcoholics are at risk for many kinds of cancer.

4 Alcohol and the Rest of Your Body

Another organ to which alcohol does incredibly disgusting things is the pancreas. This means that you probably want to know what your pancreas is and what it does.

Good questions. The pancreas is a special organ right near the liver and stomach that makes a whole assortment of important chemicals for your body. If it weren't for your beautiful white, healthy pancreas, you wouldn't be able to eat cheeseburgers, run 100 yards, or grow healthy and tall! Your pancreas makes enzymes that help you digest fat and protein, as well as the hormones insulin and glucagon, which regulate the level of sugar in your blood. People without working pancreases—just like people without

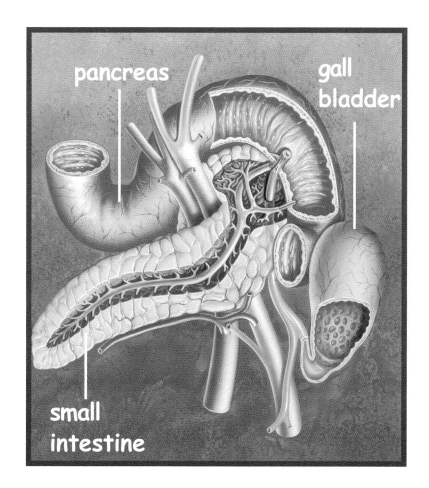

pancreas

gall bladder

small intestine

working livers, hearts, and brains—can die really quickly without proper medical treatment.

Alcohol can cause a terrible disease known as pancreatitis—a sick, swollen pancreas. A pancreas with this disease often turns black or greenish and sometimes is surrounded by lots of blood, fluid, and greenish pus. People with pancreatitis get awful belly pain and fevers. Sometimes it takes weeks or months before they are able

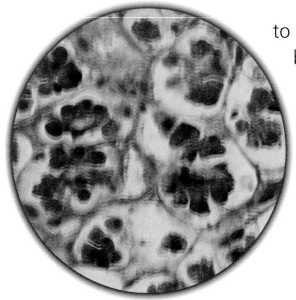

Alcohol can cause pancreatitis, the inflammation of the pancreas.

to eat again. They have to be fed through a special intravenous (IV) tube that drips nutrients directly into their blood. Can you imagine not eating for six months?

ALCOHOL AND YOUR BRAIN

You probably know a little bit about the brain—it's that mushy gray organ that is helping you read this book! Well, your brain is pretty important to you. (Think of all the fun stuff you would miss out on if you didn't have one!)

Alcohol, of course, messes up that lovely brain. After one or two drinks, your brain is just a little bit abnormal, and you may start to feel a little bit drunk.

Add another three or four drinks, and the parts of the brain that let you walk and talk start to act funny. You try to stand up, and you wobble. You try to talk clearly, but all the words come out garbled.

Add another ten drinks, and the important brain-center that tells you if you're awake and breathing can stop working completely. If your brain stops telling you to breathe, you stop breathing. If you stop breathing, you die. That's how people die from drinking too much.

Sometimes alcohol messes up people's memories. Blackouts happen when people forget chunks of time while they were drinking. Many binge drinkers get blackouts. They can be very scary because people can realize that they are "missing" periods of time, but they have no idea where they were, what they did, or who they were with during that time. How would you like to wake up in a strange place with no memory of what you did the night before? There have been many cases of people committing crimes, even murder, while in the middle of blackouts and having absolutely no recollection of what they have done.

Alcohol can kill specific parts of the brain. One of the weirdest things that happens to alcoholics is a disease with a tricky name: Wernicke-Korsakoff syndrome. This is a disease that happens only to alcoholics, and it makes them lose their memory completely! If you had a conversation with one of these poor people, and then you came back ten minutes later, he or she would have no memory

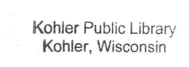

of the conversation. Imagine having no memory of what you did just ten minutes ago! People with this disease usually also tremble and have a hard time making precise movements. Other alcoholics end up with a breakdown of the cerebellum, the part of the brain that controls walking and balance. Alcohol sure can pickle people's brains!

Binge drinkers—people who drink occasionally but heavily—can suffer from memory loss and foggy thinking for a long time after they drink. Fortunately, these problems get better a few days or weeks after the drinker abstains from (stops) drinking alcohol.

ALCOHOL AND YOUR BLOOD AND HEART

Your blood and your heart can also get in trouble from too much alcohol. Your blood spreads oxygen and nutrients around the body, and your heart is the engine that pumps your blood around. When you drink alcohol, it acts as a poison for the cells living in your bone marrow that make blood cells. Also, since alcoholics usually don't eat a good diet and get the nutrients they need for healthy blood, blood forms slowly. That means that people who drink alcohol can get anemia (low blood levels), which makes them feel tired.

Alcoholism also makes the immune cells (white blood cells) in your blood work poorly. That increases your chances of getting infections. Sometimes when people drink too much, they vomit, and because they are unconscious, they breathe some

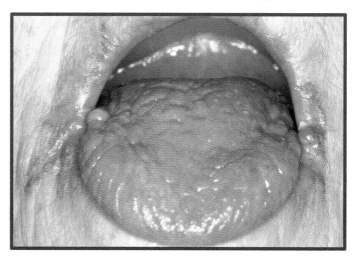

Anemia, or a deficiency of iron in the blood-stream, can cause a red, swollen tongue. The cracked, inflamed appearance of the tongue shown here indicates that this person has developed a blood disorder.

of their own vomit right into their lungs. This can cause terrible pneumonia (lung infections).

Heavy drinking can cause heart disease. The kind of heart disease that alcohol causes—cardiomyopathy—is an illness of the heart muscle. Instead of being thick and strong, the heart muscle gets stretched out and flabby like a soggy piece of pizza. Then the heart starts to work very badly. People feel weak and tired, start to huff and puff, and see their legs get swollen with extra fluid because of their sick heart. In the long term, cardiomyopathy can be fatal.

ALCOHOL AND THE REST OF YOUR BODY

Alcohol is a poison, and it can affect different parts of the body in different people. Some binge drinkers wake up the day after they drink alcohol with very painful and swollen muscles because their muscles have been poisoned and are dying. All of this muscle damage can lead to kidney damage—and your body needs your kidneys to stay alive!

Other gross things that alcohol can do include:

- Alcohol can make you vomit, and too much vomiting can rip your esophagus open.

- Alcohol can make men's testicles and women's ovaries shrink, and it can make men grow big breasts!

- Alcohol can make the blood vessels on your face expand, so that they look like big red spiders.

- Alcohol can make your fingers curl up permanently.

Are you grossed out yet? Not surprising: Alcohol does horrifying things to drinkers! Think about all of the organs that get messed up by alcohol. But when some people drink alcohol, they hurt not just their own bodies but other people's bodies,too. Check this out:

ALCOHOL AND YOUR BABY!

If you thought that alcohol was just poisonous to the people who drink it, think again! How about those babies?

Drinking alcohol can make women less able to have babies—it is harder for them to become pregnant, and they often lose their pregnancies before their babies are ready to be born.

When a pregnant woman drinks alcohol, she and her baby get drunk. Can you imagine a drunk baby? Not a very cute idea, huh? Well, when babies get drunk, terrible things can happen. Some of these children can be born with what is called fetal alcohol syndrome, which can result in such problems as mental retardation, seizures, learning disabilities, and long-term behavioral difficulties. Sometimes the skin around their eyes looks abnormal, their teeth are small, their hearts can be defective, and their joints don't work properly. Sometimes they come out with a very small head.

5 Alcohol Withdrawal and Treatment

When alcoholics stop drinking (because they run out of money, because they get too weak, or because their families try to protect them), they can get very sick. Their bodies are so used to alcohol that they get sick without it. This is called withdrawal. The worst part of withdrawal, which doesn't happen to everyone, is the shaking and the mental problems, called delirium tremens (DT, or DTs, for short). It is called delirium because people become delirious (confused and partly asleep), and tremens because people tremble. People with the DTs often hallucinate (imagine things that aren't really there).

So alcoholics can get sick from drinking and sick from not drinking? Alcohol is a poison, but it's an addictive poison. Alcoholics get so used to having alcohol in their system that they get very sick when they stop for even a little while. Withdrawal is very dangerous. So how can alcoholics ever become healthy again?

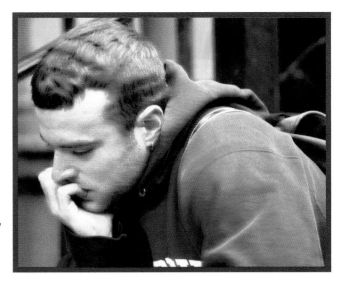

The easiest way to keep people from becoming alcoholics is to stop them from drinking in the first place! Learn what alcohol can do to your body. The more you know, the less likely you are to let alcohol get you in trouble.

GETTING WELL

Treating alcoholics is tough. There are a few medicines that make people feel sick when they drink alcohol, but they don't work very well. The main reason they fail is that people stop taking them! Some other medicines make alcoholics less interested in alcohol, but they do not seem to work very well, either. Many alcoholics and binge drinkers do not want to keep drinking and wish they could stop—but they can't. They're addicted. It is not a glamorous or a healthy lifestyle. The two main treatment methods for alcoholism are detoxification centers and twelve-step or self-help programs, of which the most famous is Alcoholics Anonymous.

Detoxification centers are special centers where alcoholics are treated for their alcoholism and withdrawal. Alcoholic patients usually stay for several days or weeks, although some programs let the patients go home at night. Of course, drinking is not allowed. Patients talk with counselors about how to stop themselves from drinking and how to recover the jobs, families, and friends they have lost because of their drinking. Their withdrawal symptoms are treated carefully with medicines and good nutrition.

Unfortunately, detoxification centers do not always prevent alcoholics from drinking alcohol. Because alcohol is so addictive, for many people drinking is a major part of their life. It is important that someone who goes to a detoxification center never touch alcohol again. Recovery from any form of addiction is a lifelong process. Even a single drink can start a spiral back into alcoholism!

Alcoholics Anonymous (or AA) is a unique society that helps people stay away from drinking. Virtually every town in the United States has a local chapter of AA. Many former alcoholics attend AA meetings and are able to help each other stay sober in this way. Every member of AA is someone who is struggling with a drinking problem, and every member learns rules and guidelines that will prevent him or her from drinking again. Usually people go to meetings and discuss their problems and their feelings about drinking. By forming close relationships with other group members and talking with the group about alcoholism, many alcoholics are able to find the support and encouragement they need to stay sober. When members feel the need to drink alcohol, they have a group of friends they can turn to for help—people who know exactly what they are going through because they have been through it themselves. Although AA is not always successful, it helps many thousands of people every year from relapsing (drinking again).

This book has been all about alcohol and your body. Abusing alcohol is dangerous because it can destroy your body instantly—like Horatio's car accident, which killed two people. People who have problems with alcohol are everywhere. Do you think that you know people in your family or elsewhere that have problems related to alcohol?

Although this book concentrates on alcohol and your body, just remember what else it can do! Parents and family members who drink too much can cause problems for their children and siblings. They can be violent, abusive, irritable, reckless, or uncaring when they are drunk. They can cause big financial problems in the family by spending money on alcohol and losing job after job.

What if there's somebody in your family who has a drinking problem? What should you do?

It can be hard to help people with alcohol-related problems. Alcoholics cannot stop drinking unless they make a strong, individual effort. If they don't want to quit, it is pretty hard to make them quit!

Alcoholics can really mess up families. The most important thing is that you recognize that you are not at fault for other people's drinking problems. Talk to a school counselor, a teacher, or another trusted adult if you think that someone in your family is being abusive or threatening to you because of a problem with alcohol.

Experimenting with new things is part of growing up. Every day you learn something new about growing up (both the good things and the bad things!), about your friends at school and your family at home, about what it's like to be you! It is natural to want to try new experiences. BUT—you cannot make smart decisions about alcohol until you know the facts. It is probably a bad idea to experiment with alcohol (or any other drug) while you are still in school. People who start drinking at an early age (like

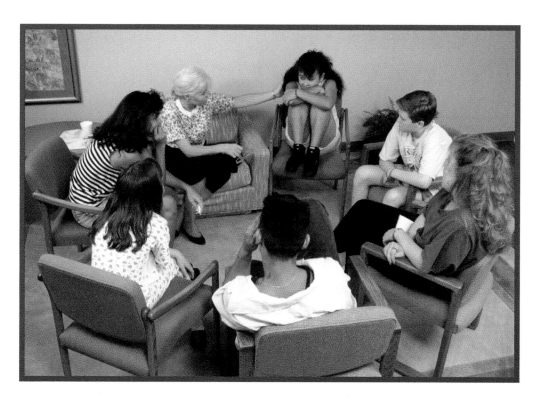

Horatio) are at a higher risk of becoming alcoholic than those who begin later in life.

If you feel pressure from your friends or other people to drink alcohol or do other drugs, remember that the important thing is not to do what your friends want you to do but to do the right thing. There are plenty of activities that don't involve alcohol and are much, much more fun. Don't risk your life on a stupid, gross, dangerous drug like alcohol.

GLOSSARY

alcohol hepatitis A disease caused by sustained and heavy drinking in which the liver swells and causes intense stomach pain, fever, and jaundice.

cirrhosis Permanent liver damage that is caused by alcoholism.

ethyl alcohol A type of drinking alcohol, also known as ethanol.

fermentation The process that makes alcohol; microorganisms turn sugar into ethanol.

pancreatitis A swollen pancreas; this disease causes the organ to change from a healthy white to black or green.

Wernicke-Korsakoff syndrome A disease that affects only alcoholics in which they lose their ability to remember recent events and conversations.

FOR MORE INFORMATION

In the United States

Al-Anon Family Groups
P.O. Box 862
Midtown Station
New York, NY 10018

Alcoholics Anonymous
P.O. Box 459
Grand Central Station
New York, NY 10163
(212) 870-3400
Web site: www.alcoholics
    anonymous.org

Chemical People Project
WQED
4802 Fifth Avenue
Pittsburgh, PA 15213

The National Clearinghouse for
    Alcohol and Drug Information
P.O. Box 2345
Rockville, MD 20847-2345
(301) 468-2600
Web site: www.health.org

National Council on Alcoholism
    and Drug Dependence
12 West 21st Street
New York, NY 10010
(800) 622-2255
e-mail: national@NCADD.org

Youth Crisis Hot Line
(800) 448-4663

In Canada

Alcohol and Drug Dependency
    Information and Counseling
    Services (ADDICS)
24711/2 Portage Avenue, Suite 2
Winnipeg, MB R3J ON 6
(204) 942-4730

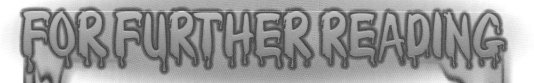

FOR FURTHER READING

Clayton, Lawrence. *Coping with a Drug-Abusing Parent.* New York: Rosen Publishing Group, 1995.

Fishman, Ross. *Alcohol and Alcoholism.* New York: Chelsea House, 1986.

Grosshandler, Janet. *Coping with Drinking and Driving.* New York: Rosen Publishing Group, 1997.

Hyde, Margaret O., and Bruce G. Hyde. *Know About Drugs.* New York: McGraw Hill, 1979.

Madison, Arnold. *Drugs and You.* New York: Julian Messner, 1972.

Ryan, Elizabeth A. *Straight Talk About Drugs and Alcohol.* New York: Facts on File, 1989.

Shuker, Nancy. *Everything You Need to Know About an Alcoholic Parent.* New York: Rosen Publishing Group, 1998.

Taylor, Barbara. *Everything You Need to Know About Alcohol.* New York: Rosen Publishing Group, 1996.

Vogler, Roger E., and Wayne Bartz. *Teenagers and Alcohol: When Saying No Isn't Enough.* Philadelphia: The Charles Press, 1992.

INDEX

CREDITS

About the Author

Theresa Anne Booley is a freelance writer with diverse interests. She has live and traveled in Malaysia, France, Senegal, Alaska and Ecuador, and is currently a medical student at Harvard Medical School in Boston, Massachusetts. In her spare time, she enjoys playing guitar in her band, Vynyng Phayze, reading literature, playing basketball and taking advanced graduate courses in the preparation of Middle Eastern cuisine.

Photo Credits

Series Design and Layout

Laura Murawski